Be FIT

Foundations for Integrative Faith and Fitness from the "Be Well" Collection

Dr. Eugene R. Furnace

BE FIT ROUTINES

A library of integrative faith and fitness routines

GENERAL

Body Basics
> *An introductory routine that includes a total body workout and stretches.*

Manhood
> *Faith and fitness building routine highlighting scriptures and postures of men.*

Womanhood
> *Faith and fitness building routine highlighting scriptures and postures of women.*

WINNING

Affirmation
> *Low-intensity routine with encouraging, forward-moving scriptures.*

Breakthrough
> *Moderate-intensity routine seeking a breakthrough based on the cross.*

Warfare
> *High-intensity routine through spiritual and physical battle positions.*

AWAKING

Focus
> *Movements through scriptures, body positions, and emotions that guide the mind to focus.*

Clarity
> *Movements through scriptures, body positions, thoughts, emotions, and desires to seek clarity.*

Direction
> *Movements through scriptures, body positions, and desires to acquire direction.*

RESTORING

Peace
> *Movements through scriptures, body positions, and desires to guide emotions and thoughts to peace.*

Rest
> *Movements through scriptures and body positions to induce rest.*

Release
> *Movements through scriptures, body positions, thoughts, emotions, and desires to release.*

CONTENTS

ACKNOWLEDGMENTS

Professor Denise Bednarczyk for guiding me to research-informed practices and teaching me to develop fitness programs that are effective and fun.

Adrien Albert, of Live Physical, for being a great personal trainer and helping me reach my personal fitness goals.

Karla Andrade, of Verus Health and Fitness, for bouncing ideas around and being a great supporter of health and fitness in my life.

ABOUT THE AUTHOR

Dr. Eugene R. Furnace is a health services provider and clinical pastoral counselor. He has completed degrees in multiple fields of study, including behavioral health, psychology, kinesiology, health, and wellness. Dr. Furnace has served as a consultant and trainer for many healthcare professionals, conferences, and organizations. He has also been a professor in undergraduate and graduate studies at various universities. Just as with his "Biblically Based and Scientifically Supported" approach to Be Well, Dr. Furnace posits the interconnectedness of Biblical truth and scientific fact throughout the human experience. This philosophy is demonstrated in his clinical practice, ministry, and personal walk with God.

1 INTRODUCTION

For many people, time seems to be an enemy. They fight against time because it is limited, always moving forward, and never enough of it in a day to do all the things they want. Work, school, children, relationships, goals, and many more things place a demand on time. No matter what is done, even when nothing is done, time is still spent. People create lists, maintain calendars, set reminders, and try various tools and activities to maximize, validate, and control time. Sometimes it works. Sometimes it is only a reminder of the things left undone.

Nonetheless, they contend with time, for it is the natural, objective measure life.

The most common discussion I have with people about morning routines is the time crunch. They want to workout, but must get the children ready for school. They want to complete a morning devotional, but must prepare for work. Notice how the wants are outranked by the musts. In many instances, for many decisions, we do what we must do and forfeit what we want to do. This is understandable, yet hardly acceptable. We give so much of ourselves away to the things required to "make it" in life that we struggle or neglect giving ourselves to things that help us live and thrive.

A simple, yet profound, prayer of John is written in 3 John 2:2. John prayed that you may prosper and be in good health, that you may do well in every way of life, both spiritually and naturally. This encompasses the entire E.M.P.I.R.E. of health and wellness, not just the must dos or have-to-dos. I echo the prayer of John and desire that you achieve well-being Environmentally, Mentally, Physically, Intellectually, Relationally, and Emotionally (E.M.P.I.R.E.). I, too, pray that you may prosper in all ways of life! This is why I have written the "Be Well" series, so we can progressively increase our understanding of health and wellness and practically prosper on our journeys. Yes, I say we and include myself because these are revelations and practices in my life that I research, implement, measure, and then share.

I have struggled with a morning routine that includes all the things I want to accomplish at the start of my day, particularly some spiritual discipline that gives time to God (praying, meditating, studying, reading) and some workout regimen that gives time to physical health (heart, muscles, bones, lungs). Many days, during my cardio work (treadmill, bicycle, elliptical, etcetera), I listen to sermons or Christian music to feed my spirit while I work my body. One day, I was doing a core workout and the position of my body brought to mind a spiritual position. I began to think (meditate) on that spiritual principle as I continued through the workout. After the workout was over, I realized that with a little ingenuity and insight I was able to accomplish wants without forsaking the musts by integrating activities (a spiritual discipline and a workout regimen). This integration increased the use of my time, so I was able to move to other activities feeling accomplished!

What if you were able to "kill two birds with one stone" and accomplish a morning exercise and devotion? What if you were able effectively to combine two of your wants into one time block so you no longer had to sacrifice either of them? What if you could integrate your faith with your fitness?

That is the teaching of this book! Be FIT (where FIT means Faith In Training) provides basic instructions for integrating faith and fitness into one routine that can be done in the morning, midday, evening, or any time you want to dedicate minutes to faith and fitness. The exercises and scriptures in the Be FIT library of integrated faith and fitness routines have been carefully chosen and paired so the body and soul (thoughts, emotions, and desires) move harmoniously through the routine while drawing on Scriptures to direct flow. All of the exercises can be done at home, in a park, in an office space, or any other environment with space to move (internally and externally) freely. There are no equipment or weight requirements. You may want a mat simply to define your space and/or provide comfort, but it is not necessary. You can also use a large towel to define your space.

Included in this book are discussions of physical fitness principles and foundational processes of select spiritual disciplines. It should be noted that to achieve maximal health and wellness in each domain of well-being (to build your E.M.P.I.R.E. of Health and Wellness), you will have to give dedicated time to each domain individually. Integrated approaches are great time-savers and absolutely beneficial. They do not take away from the need sometimes to just pray, or just be present with another, or just have a great leg day at the gym.

Also included in this book is the Body Basics routine that can be adapted to any faith and/or fitness level. It is a total body workout that includes stretches and body weight training. The Body Basics routine serves as an introductory routine to integrating faith and fitness and can be dialed down or amped up depending on how much you want to do. So, let's Be FIT!

2 BODY BASICS

To complete this routine, you will need approximately 25 to 30 minutes. This can be done any time during the day or night. The Body Basics routine includes warm-up stretching and twenty minutes of a total body workout. Scriptures have been paired with the stretches. Stretches may be repeated at the end of the routine to help cool the body down.

This routine is scalable for various faith and fitness levels. Regardless of fitness level, it is recommended that you start at the beginner faith level so that you are able to focus on form (safety) while learning the skill of integration. You need to train your body to complete the moves safely and properly so your mind has the ability to shift its forward attention to the Scripture.

To scale the routine for faith, considering the following:

- Beginner faith: Read and verbally (aloud) recite the Scripture while completing the stretch. The rehearsal (or recitation) of the Scripture will help you write the Word on your heart, or memorize it.

- Intermediate faith: During the cycles of the stretch, alternate reading the Scripture and thinking of an event in your life when that Scripture proved true or helpful. In doing this, you fortify your history with God's Word being true in your own life.

- Advanced faith: Read the Scripture and think about how it connects with other Scriptures and applies to your life. In doing this, you formulate a systematic theological meditation.

To scale the routine for fitness, consider the following:

- Beginner fitness: Focus on proper form and moderately complete rounds 1 and 2 by cutting the repetitions for each exercise in half (where 20 is noted, do 10; where 40 is noted, do 20).
- Intermediate fitness: Focus on proper form and complete as many rounds as possible in 20 minutes.
- Advanced fitness: Focus on proper form and complete as many rounds as possible in 20 minutes as supersets, pairing the exercises from each round in the order they are listed (i.e., squats/lunges, pushups/hip hinges,

bridges/scissor kicks, and crunches/glute kickbacks).

Once you have the routine down, additional variations can be applied. You may want to consider using it as a high-intensity workout. In doing so, the Body Basics routine may be used for cardiorespiratory gains. You may also want to consider using the routine as a muscle conditioning workout by slowing down the exercise movements to increase muscle activation for stability. In what ever ways you modify the routine to meet your faith and fitness needs, always practice safety first.

NOTE: Consult with your primary care provider before beginning a fitness regimen. Safety and proper form are more important than speed and high counts. Doing less safely is better than doing more unsafely.

BODY BASICS ROUTINE

Time: Approximately 25 to 30 minutes

Intensity: Scalable to individual needs and preferences.

Instructions: Start with stretches to warm the body up. After completing stretches, move on to rounds. Complete round 1, then round 2, then round 1, then round 2, continuing to alternate rounds for twenty (20) minutes. Stretches may be repeated after 20 minutes of rounds to cool the body down.

In general, dynamic stretches may be useful to warm the body up and static stretches may be useful to cool the body down. For more on each, see "Flexibility Training" in Chapter 3 Fitness Foundations. To convert alternating dynamic stretches to static stretches in the Body Basics routine, stretch and hold each side once for up to 20 seconds.

Stretches

Time (repetitions)	Movement (physical activity)	Meditation (spiritual activity)
12 repetitions (alternating; 6 for each side; stretch, recite Scripture, then swltch sides)	Side Stretch with Overhead Reach	I lift up holy hands without anger and doubt. *I Timothy 2:8*
12 repetitions (reach for toes, recite Scripture, release, and then repeat)	Sitting Toe Touch	I set my heart on God and stretch my hands to Him. *Job 11:13*
12 repetitions (alternating; 6 for each side; stretch, recite Scripture, then switch sides)	Truck Twist	I release the things behind me to focus on things ahead. *Philippians 3:13*
12 repetitions (gently press knees toward ground, recite Scripture, release, and then repeat)	Sitting Inner Thigh Stretch	I press toward the goal in Jesus Christ. *Philippians 3:14*

Exercises

Time (repetitions)	Movement (physical activity)	Primary Muscle Group
ROUND 1		
20	Squats	Legs
20	Standard Pushups	Chest
20	Bridges	Buttocks
40	Bicycle Crunches	Core
ROUND 2		
20	Lunges	Legs
20	Hip Hinges	Back
40	Scissor Kicks	Core
40	Glute Kickbacks	Buttocks

Remember, the Body Basics routine is an introductory routine to jump-start or enhance your integration of faith and fitness. For additional routines, consider the Be FIT library.

3 FITNESS FOUNDATIONS

The fitness industry has blossomed greatly over decades and has branched into many academic and professional disciplines. Fitness is now a broad term employed with many applications and may reference various concepts from appearance (looking fit), to lifestyle (living fit), to nutrition (eating fit), to medicine (prescribing fit). In all the shades and variations of fitness, however, there remains a necessary constant, which is physical activity. Fitness, at its core and through its branches, is about movement of the body and the ability to increase or improve movement of the body. In this discussion, we will look at fitness from the perspective of physical exercise that contributes to overall health and wellness.

Yes, exercise is more than just getting a summer beach body or fitting into your skinny jeans. Physical exercise carries with it immense implications for your entire E.M.P.I.R.E. of Health and Wellness. Most notably, physical exercise has been positively correlated with heart, mental, emotional, metabolic, and social health. Lack of physical activity and exercise (hypokinesis) is an independent risk factor for the origin and progression of several chronic medical diseases such as heart disease, diabetes (specifically Type II), and obesity. Additionally, improvements in heart health, mood (depression and anxiety), and weight loss are gained with adequate physical activity and exercise. Here, again, we see interplay and connectedness between the dimensions of well-being.

Physical exercise is not only scientifically supported, it is found in Scripture many times. Physical activity was so common in Bible times that just as stories are told of agricultural work to convey spiritual truths, so are stories told of athletic work to communicate spiritual principles. For example, Paul writes to the church in Corinth:

> Don't you realize that everyone who runs in a race runs to win, but only one runner gets the prize? Run like them, so that you can win. Everyone who enters an athletic contest goes into strict training. They do it to win a temporary crown, but we do it to win one that will be permanent. So I run—but not without a clear goal ahead of me. So I box—but not as if I were just shadow boxing. Rather, I toughen my body with punches and make it my slave so that I will not be disqualified after I have spread the Good News to others. (I Corinthians 9:24-27 GW)

Clearly, physical exercise played a role in society then, and physical exercise has a significant role in society now. Moreover, your body is a temple of the Holy Spirit whom you received from God (I Corinthians 6:9). Taking care of His temple is important. This verse of Scripture informs the Christian reader you do not belong to yourself, so your body is not yours to do whatever and however you want with it. You, and your body, belong to God. I suggest you take care of God's property!

A well-rounded physical exercise program is multifaceted. For the best benefits, you want a program that properly highlights cardiorespiratory functioning (to improve heart and lung capacity), musculoskeletal functioning (to improve muscle and bone performance), and joint functioning (to improve range of motion). Here are considerations, or rules, to know when engaging in an exercise regimen. Remember, "Whoever enters an athletic competition wins the prize only when playing by the rules" (II Timothy 2:5 GW).

Safety. Consult with your healthcare provider before beginning an exercise program. This seems unnecessary to many people, but there is good reason to speak with your primary care provider before engaging in rigorous activity that will place demands on your heart, lungs, metabolism, bones, and muscles. Especially if you have a known diagnosis or condition, it is very important to discuss the dos and don'ts with your healthcare provider, and then share that information with your personal trainer or exercise physiologist (if you decide to work with a fitness professional).

During physical activity or any specific exercise, physical pain is not gain. There may be soreness after strength and conditioning routines. That is normal and will pass in intensity and frequency as you continue to exercise. During an exercise, you may feel resistance, have to exert more-than-usual force, and/or push yourself to finish, but do not hurt yourself. Feelings of pain during exercise could be symptomatic of an underlying health matter, associated with improper form, the use of excessive weight, and/or other reasons that warrant stopping the exercise and seeking professional, maybe medical, attention and assistance.

Progress Measures. Use various assessments to track and measure your progress. The mirror and/or scale alone are not sufficient indicators of your improvements. The following are ideas to help you monitor and measure your progress.

- You may use measuring tape to record the before and after circumference of thighs, biceps, midsection, and other body areas in which you are trying to lose weight or gain muscle. For example, you may start with 14 inch biceps, gain muscle, and improve to 15 inch biceps.

- You may use the distance you walk on a treadmill in a certain time period to measure increased cardiorespiratory capacity. For example, you start walking 1 mile in 15 minutes and improve to walking 1 mile in 10 minutes.

- If you are more time bound, you may still use the distance you walk on a treadmill in a certain time period. For example, you start walking 1 mile in 20 minutes and improve to walking 2 miles in 20 minutes.

- If you are at home using the Body Basics routine in this book, you can measure your progress by how many rounds you are able to complete in 20 minutes. For example, you start being able to complete 2 rounds in 20 minutes and improve to completing 4 rounds in 20 minutes.

- For those who are strength training, you may use the amount of weight you are able to lift/press/pull to measure muscle strength. For example, you may start bench pressing 100 pounds and improve to bench pressing 150 pounds.

- For those who are muscle conditioning at home using body weight, you may use the number of repetitions you can accomplish prior to failure to measure muscle endurance. For example, you may start being able to complete 20 pushups before you fatigue and improve to completing 35 pushups before fatigue.

There are many ways to monitor and measure your progress and improvement. Relying on a scale and/or mirror alone does not give you objective and accurate indicators of how great you are doing on your fitness journey and how much you have accomplished.

Cardiorespiratory Training. Because of the overall health and performance benefits, cardiorespiratory training is largely considered the most important fitness element. Increasing muscle mass without increasing cardiorespiratory endurance does not lead to total body health and wellness. In fact, the body's ability naturally to build muscle can be negatively affected without building cardiorespiratory capacity.

To receive optimal benefits from cardiorespiratory exercise, aim for at least 30 minutes of moderate to intense physical activity once a day 4 to 5 days each week. This can be varied to something like 45 minutes 3 days each week or 20 minutes 7 days each week depending on fitness level and goals. Be advised, however, the best range for the average person is believed to be somewhere between 30 and 45 minutes of moderate-intense cardiorespiratory training regularly and frequently throughout the week. This 30- to 45-minute range of cardiorespiratory training may promote good heart conditioning, enhance caloric and fat burn, release positive body chemicals (such as neurotransmitters, neuropeptides, and hormones), and avoid an increased creation of harmful atoms in the body (such as free radicals).

High-intensity cardiorespiratory training has great fat-burning benefits and requires less time during the workout because the after-workout burn is greater with intense training than with moderate training. It is strongly recommended to consult with your healthcare provider prior to engaging in any fitness routine, and especially a high-intensity routine. You may want to discuss with your healthcare provider the use of antioxidant supplements or dietary improvements to combat the increased free radicals produced by intense workouts and ensure you fuel your body for the intensity.

Muscle Training. Perform weightlifting exercises, as appropriate, using the full range of motion to avoid irregular muscle and joint development. In general, lower weight at higher repetitions (8-12) tone and increase endurance while higher weight at lower repetitions (4-6) build mass. Due to the law of diminished returns, for the average person, it is recommended not to exceed 15 repetitions. Muscle training has two components: strength and endurance. While big gains in mass are better accomplished using weights, both muscular strength and muscular endurance can be improved with at-home exercises and body weight.

Weight lifting has a bit of a science to it, if you will, that when followed properly produces safe movements and effective outcomes. Generally speaking, you can use a 2:2 timing when lifting weights. That is, 2 seconds of muscle contraction (lifting, pressing, or pulling) and 2 seconds of muscle relaxation (returning to starting position or beginning point of next movement). During contraction and relaxation, the muscle is working so do not think of relaxation as easy. Relaxation is just the word used here to make the concept easy to understand and apply. Think of a standard bicep curl. Use a 1, 2 count to lift the weight while contracting your bicep muscles as you move the dumbbell up to your shoulder followed by a 1, 2 count to lower the weight while relaxing your bicep muscles as you straighten your arm and return to the starting position. Lift count 1, 2. Lower count 1, 2. There are variations to the timing of weight lifting (1:1, 2:4, and others), so do not get stuck on 2:2 if you are working with a fitness professional who directs you otherwise. The 2:2 timing is a decent start for beginners or returners after an absence from weight training because it promotes a slow, controlled movement.

Breathing is critical during muscle training. It is a natural reaction to hold your breath when handling a heavy object or attempting to exert force. Do not do it! Use your knowledge of timing to aid in your breathing. Remember 2:2? Lift count 1, 2. Lower count 1, 2. Your breathing can follow the same pattern! Take a breath—inhale—before you begin the exercise movement to fill your body with air (oxygen). Exhale while lifting and count 1, 2. Inhale while lowering and count 1, 2. Exhale as you contract (lift, press, or pull) so the pressure in your body from exerting force has an escape. This is useful, for example, in reducing hernias due to holding your breath and giving the internal body pressure no external release.

Inhale as you relax (return to starting position). This helps recharge your cells with oxygen in preparation for the next contraction (lift, press, or pull).

Flexibility Training. The best outcomes occur with daily stretches that are held no more than 60 cumulative seconds per stretch. Perform appropriate stretches for the entire body to the point of stretch or tension, but not pain. Pain could be an indicator of various complications, including hyperextension (over extending) of the joint. Yes, you may experience tightness in your muscles and joints that require some extra effort to increase flexibility. Working through tightness is not to be confused with self-inflicting pain. Generally, stretch to the point of tightness and maybe slightly beyond. You may feel some discomfort. Your muscles may shake. If you feel pain, stop immediately. There may be exceptions to the feeling of pain during rehabilitative stretching, and in this scenario, and all others, follow the direction(s) of your healthcare provider.

Breathing while stretching is very important. Both static (still) and dynamic (moving) stretches have a rhythm. During a static stretch, as you inhale, you release just a little from the full stretch and then exhale to go deeper into the stretch. Grand movements and a full release of the stretch are not part of the static stretch. Just a slight release, enough to allows your body to rise and fill with air. During a dynamic stretch, as you inhale, you may fully release the stretch and then reengage as you exhale. Dynamic stretching can be useful in warming the body up for exercise and static stretching can be useful in cooling the body down after exercise (and reducing soreness or tightness from training).

Nutrition. A change in physical activity may trigger a change in the nutritional needs of the body. Starting physical activity for the first time, or after an absence from training, definitely requires a review of nutritional needs for your body. A balanced diet is best, regardless of fitness goals. The body needs appropriate (not excessive) proteins, appropriate (not restricted) carbohydrates, and appropriate (not avoided) fats. To develop an appropriate diet for your fitness goals, consult with a nutrition professional.

4 FAITH FOUNDATIONS

Spiritual disciplines exist in virtually every faith group. They are the practices by which spiritual formation, maturity, or growth may occur. Spiritual disciplines are encouraged by leaders in the church, and have been practiced throughout history by followers and seekers of God (including Hebraic/Jewish and Christian persons). Although spiritual disciplines can be practiced in particular ways per people group, there are some universal points to certain spiritual disciplines.

The term discipline in the phrase "spiritual discipline" can be confusing. Discipline can be used to mean a branch of study or knowledge, such as an academic discipline. Discipline can mean corrective action, such as an organization's disciplinary policy. Discipline may also be used to mean training someone to obey rules and behave in specified manners, such as disciplining a child. Regardless of use, the word discipline suggests there is some consistency of effort required to engage the practice—be it studying, correcting, or training. All three of these uses are applicable to spiritual disciplines. Moreover, all spiritual disciplines require consistency of effort to be optimally effective in spiritual health.

Although there are many spiritual disciplines and exhaustive lists of what they may or may not include, we will focus on two: engaging the Word and meditating. By focusing on these two spiritual disciplines, we are better able to understand how to integrate them into our fitness routines.

Engaging the Word. There are two specific practices we can apply here. First is hearing the Word, and second is memorizing the Word. For many years, people did not have access to the written Word of God we now know as the Bible. Even today, there are individuals and people groups who may not be able to read, may not have access to Scripture in their language, or may not be able to purchase a Bible. God does not hold such technicalities against people. Besides, the Bible itself teaches that people during the early church listened to Jesus's, John's, and Paul's sermons. Furthermore, faith comes by hearing (Romans 10:17). So while some place an emphasis on reading the Word, I encourage you to engage the Word in a manner that is accessible and achievable to you as an individual with your personal circumstances and preferences in mind.

If you are reading this book, then you are able to read the Word. Reading Scripture, thereby, is an accessible and achievable means for you to engage God's Word. Great! That makes the process of integrating faith and fitness using the tools in this book realistic for you! It also gives you a double-edged sword, if you will. If you can read the Word, then you may be able to speak and subsequently hear the Word. Reciting a Scripture aloud allows you to process it twice: 1) the cognitive process to speak it and 2) the cognitive process to hear it. If you do not or cannot recite the Scripture aloud, reading and reciting it in your mind also activates multiple cognitive processes.

Each Be FIT routine, including the Body Basics routine in this book, is constructed to guide you through reading and reciting Scripture with a paired movement that bodily reinforces or illustrates the Scripture. It does not, however, stop there.

We are to take the words of God to heart and keep them in mind (Deuteronomy 11:18). Words of wisdom are to be written on the tablets of our hearts (Proverbs 7:3). There are other Scriptures that share the sentiment of memorizing God's Word so that we keep it with us and allow it to guide us. Only hearing or reading the Word is not enough! We are to be doers of the Word, not just hearers (James 1:22). It is not practical to walk about with a Bible in hand and flip through pages of Scripture, or read through search results for us Bible app users, every time something comes up in life. Memorizing the Word is useful for daily living and decision-making.

One of the ways we can engage the Word—hearing, reading, and/or memorizing—is through meditation. Meditation involves recitation, or rehearsal, of the Word you have heard or read. One tool that may be useful in efforts to memorize the Word, which can also be employed during meditation, is elaborative rehearsal.

Elaborative rehearsal is the process of linking new information with data you already know. In doing so, you may increase the quantity and quality of retrieval cues, which would make recalling the new information more effective. When meditating on the Word, you can use elaborative rehearsal to link the Scripture to an experience. By doing so, you connect several cues (thoughts, emotions, memories, words, etcetera) to the Scripture, which may improve your ability to recall, or remember, that Scripture. Be advised to link the Scripture to appropriate experiences. This is not the time to link "Vengeance is mine" (Romans 12:19) with the time you *accidentally* spilled food in your friend's car because they ordered the wrong meal for you. Remember, God's Word is holy. Treat it accordingly.

There are other ways to utilize elaborative rehearsal during meditation, but using experiences is maybe the most universal since we all have them. This is an example of how using elaborative rehearsal during meditation on the Word may be: The Scripture is Romans 12:17 (GW), "Don't pay people back with evil for the evil they do to you." The experience is the coworker who falsely reported your attendance to upper management. By linking this Scripture with that experience, you create several reference points in your mind that can be used for current and, ideally, future recall. Another example is as follows: The Scripture is Philippians 4:6 (GW), "Never worry about anything. But in every situation let God know what you need in prayers and requests while giving thanks." The experience is the memory of worry when you received bad medical news and the healing God gave you anyhow. By linking this Scripture with that experience, you reinforce your faith that worry is not necessary when you have God on your side and enhance your ability to remember that Scripture because it matches your experience.

The book of Joshua records a very direct command and connection between engaging the Word and meditation.

This book of the law shall not depart from your mouth, but you shall meditate on it day and night, so that you may be careful to do according to all that is written in it; for then you will make your way prosperous, and then you will have success (Joshua 1:8 NASB).

Meditation. Meditation is not necessarily a blank or empty state of mind. It is not shutting your mind off so that you do not think of anything. Quite the opposite, especially in the initial stages of learning how to meditate, meditation requires focus and cognitive engagement at levels sometimes higher than normal. Meditation may involve intense focus on a specific thought or phrase and requires concentration. To aid with that concentration, meditation can include a low, repetitive, mumbling of a phrase or word (sometimes referred to as chanting).

Christian meditation can involve reciting Scripture while occupying one's mind with the repetition of Scripture, God's works, or some other determined focal point. However, the options for content on which we can meditate are almost limitless. From the Psalms, we learn that we can meditate on:

    the Lord's works (in creation and in our lives),

    the Lord's precepts (principles and general rules),

    the Lord's statutes (laws and commandments),

    the glorious splendor of the Lord's majesty (His greatness, dignity, authority), and the Lord's Word (the written Word in Scripture and the spoken word, as by a preacher or prophet).

We must include Scripture in our meditative practices, but Scripture is not the only thing we can use during meditation. The love of a relationship, the virtue of holiness, the splendor of nature, the beauty of art and music, and anything praiseworthy is also meditation worthy (see Philippians 4:8-9).

Scripture pairings with dynamic stretches and isotonic exercises can be done and is part of certain Be FIT routines. The deeper you want to go into your meditation, the more you may consider positions with little movement so you exercise and meditate safely with good form of body and mind.

Pairing Scripture with stretches (particularly static stretches) and isometric exercises (where there is no movement of the joint or muscle; for example, a plank) may allow us to bring some meditative flow to our exercise routines. During static stretches and isometric positions, the body is held in place with minimal or no movement, which may free the mind to focus on the Lord's works, precepts, statutes, majesty, and/or Word!

Now, let's take that concept to another level and develop routines that are Word focused! Instead of bringing Scripture into your workout, your workout is built on Scripture. Let's consider the Body Basics routine in this book. Each stretch, if done correctly, positions you to express the Scripture verbally and bodily while guiding you through a release and refocus.

Side stretch with overhead reach while reciting "I lift up holy hands without anger and doubt" allows you to:

1) Inhale

2) Set your mind and body to lift holy hands overhead while leaning to the side for the stretch

3) While entering the stretch, exhale and release anger and doubt

Sitting toe touch while reciting "I set my heart on God and stretch my hands to Him" allows you to:

1) Inhale

2) Set your mind and body to bend forward as you reach for your toes, bowing your heart before God to set your heart on Him

3) While entering the stretch feeling the tension/tightness in your back and/or legs wanting to pull you back, you exhale and stretch your hands to God in spite of feeling pulled back

Trunk twist while reciting "I release the things behind me to focus on things ahead" allows you to:

1) Inhale

2) Set your mind and body to turn your torso and head toward the back and figuratively see the things behind you

3) While entering the stretch, exhale and release the things behind you (remember being pulled back in the previous stretch, well here is your release from things pulling you back)

4) Return to center, signifying you are focusing on things ahead

Sitting inner thigh stretch while reciting "I press toward the goal in Jesus Christ" allows you to:

1) Inhale

2) Set your mind and body gently to press your knees toward the ground symbolizing a press toward the high calling in Christ Jesus

3) While entering the stretch, exhale and press just a little deeper symbolizing movement toward the goal

In all these movements through Scripture and stretches, you have orally and bodily expelled anger and doubt, submitted and sought God, released your past, and ended with a focus on achieving the goals God has before you. Meditating on these Scriptures means you have also strengthened your spirit through this routine. That is physical, psychological, and spiritual training in one routine! Amazing!

It does not matter where you are on your faith journey, meditation is a great practice that has spiritual, psychological, and biological benefits. If you are new to meditation, starting by following a Be FIT routine such as the Body Basic routine may be a great introduction to the spiritual discipline. If you have vast experience with meditation, then these integrative principles may illuminate new ways to employ the practice. Meditating on Scripture and maneuvering your body to support the meditative practice is an integrative wellness approach that can be done as an individual, with a family, or with a group. Additionally, if you do this with a group and share your thoughts or impressions after the routine, you are integrating another dimension of well-being by engaging in relationship!

We are all crunched for time, and we want to live and thrive, not just survive. This book provides practical tools to maximize your minutes and build your E.M.P.I.R.E. of Health and Wellness, setting you on course to prosper and be in good health with faith and fitness. Go ahead, Be FIT!